The Little A-Z Dictionary
Of
Herbal Remedies

Also By Brian B Jacques

His very popular Series of Mini-Health Books includes:

- An Easy Way To Understand Eczema and Psoriasis
- An Easy Way To Understand Stress and Depression
- An Easy Way To Understand Vitamins and Minerals
- An Easy Way To Understand Parasites, Worms, Candida, Constipation & Detoxing
- An Easy Way To Understand Crohn's Disease and IBD
- An Easy Way To Understand Body Building For Men And Women
- An Easy Way To Understand Alzheimer's Disease
- An Easy Way To Understand Herpes
- An Easy Way To Understand Parkinson's Disease
- An Easy Way To Understand Autism
- An Easy Way To Understand Fibromyalgia
- An Easy Way To Understand Your Body Systems
- An Easy Way To Understand Erectile Dysfunction
- An Easy Way To Understand Heart Disease, High Blood Pressure & Stroke
- An Easy Way To Understand Detoxing For Men & Women
- How To Lose Weight After 40
- How To Lose Weight And Maintain Your Ideal Weight Permanently
- Amino Acids & Enzymes—What Are They & Why Do You Need Them
- The Little A–Z Dictionary of Herbal Remedies
- The Magic Of Vitamins & Minerals
- Effective Methods To Stop Smoking

All these books are available as Kindle Editions (available from the Kindle Store on Amazon.com, and other countries Amazon sites where the Kindle platform is supported.) Many of these books are also available for the Barnes and Noble "Nook". In addition, all these titles will shortly be available as print editions from the Amazon website. A downloadable eBook version will also be available from the publishers website at www.wisdomforlifemedia.com

The Little A-Z Dictionary
Of
Herbal Remedies

Brian B Jacques

Wisdom For Life Media

ISBN - 13: 978-1502795175

ISBN - 10: 1502795175

Published in The United States of America

*"Education is the kindling of a flame,
not the filling of a vessel."* —Socrates

Brian B Jacques

Contents

Acknowledgment

To my wife, Tatyana, whose constant love,
presence and belief in me makes everything
possible and worthwhile.

Herbs – An Ancient, Natural Medicinal Treatment

Herbal medicine is the oldest known form of healthcare. Whether it is Western natural medicine, or Chinese, Indian or Native American, herbal combinations are used to improve the performance of various body organs.

The Chinese emperor Shen Nong (who lived around 5000BC) wrote a treatise on herbs that is still in use today. For example, Shen Nong recommended the use of Ma Huang (known as ephedra in the Western world), to treat respiratory problems. Ephedrine, extracted from ephedra, is used as a decongestant today.

In another example, King Hammurabi of Babylon (c. 1800BC) recommended the use of mint for digestive disorders. Today, peppermint is widely used to relieve nausea—especially travel sickness and vomiting.

The Middle East in particular has a rich history of herbal healing. Surviving texts from the ancient people's of Mesopotamia, Egypt and India explain with words and pictures how to use medicinal plant products, such as castor oil, linseed oil and white poppies.

During the Middle Ages, most households would have an extensive herb garden which was used to treat all the family's ailments. Home grown herbal plants were the only form of medicine available. The medicinal uses for these herbal plants were passed from generation to generation within a family by word of mouth.

In Europe, in 1649, Nicholas Culpeper wrote *A Physical Directory* and a few years later *The English Physician*. This herbal pharmacopeia was one of the first manuals that anyone could use for health care, and it is still often quoted from today.

In the nineteenth century, Western medicine as we know it today, progressed from being passed on from generation to generation where everyone who was interested had medicinal knowledge, to the realm of just a few that had a more scientific background.

This came about by scientific methods being developed to extract and synthesize active ingredients in plants to manufacture drugs. And a huge and powerful drugs industry was born.

Herbal plants contain many different compounds, active ingredients in the form of alkaloids, volatile oils, vitamins, minerals, glycosides, bioflavonoids, and other ingredients that are important in supporting a particular herbs medicinal qualities. Some of these substances have been identified, but many more have yet to be discovered.

The problem that then arises is when drugs are manufactured; an active ingredient is extracted from the natural herb and synthesized in a laboratory to emulate the natural herb's qualities. But all the other ingredients in the plant are left behind. These "other ingredients" play the role of a natural safeguard which is lost.

By comparison, it usually takes a larger amount of a whole herb, with all of its components, to reach a toxic level. The end result with the drug and its isolated active ingredient is that some of these substances can become toxic in small amounts, which can cause serious side effects from the use of these drugs.

Interestingly, watching drug commercials on TV, most of the time is taken up explaining all the side effects which the drug can cause.

Today components from plants form the basis of many medications used for such conditions as asthma, high blood pressure and heart disease to name a few.

Two examples: salicylic acid, a precursor of aspirin, was originally derived from white willow bark and the meadowsweet plant. Digitalis which is derived from the foxglove plant has been used for many years as a heart medication.

Herbs generally fall into two categories: those that grow in the wild and are called wild crafted. These are harvested where the plant grows in its natural habitat. The other is commercially grown, where a greater control over quality and growing conditions can be exercised.

Herbal products are available in several forms: liquid, tablets, capsules, tinctures, teas, salves, ointments, fresh, or as dried plant parts. Some are supplied as single herbs while others are made into combinations to treat a specific condition.

Capsules and Tablets

The herb is ground into a very fine powder and then either inserted into a capsule or pressed into a tablet form. Generally, herbs in capsules and tablets are less potent than tinctures or extracts. Additionally, read the label to make sure no fillers have been added. Fillers could be either natural or synthetic.

Extracts

Extracts can be made with alcohol like tinctures, or glycerin or water can be used. Like tinctures the herb is in a concentrated form and is easily assimilated by the body. The only way to tell what method has been used is to read the label.

Lozenges

Lozenges are often sucked to ward off the effects of a cold or cough, or they may be used as a decongestant. Many are fortified with vitamin C. Read the label to make sure they are not coated with refined sugar or an artificial sweetener.

Ointments, Salves, and Rubs

There are many products available in your health food store or on the Internet to treat burns, wounds, skin rashes and insect bites, or as heat producing herbs to treat sprains, pulled muscles or to relax muscle aches.

Teas

A huge selection of herbal teas is available either from your health food store, supermarket or on the Internet. Herbal teas take several forms from being relaxing, comforting or having medicinal properties. They come either as loose tea or in tea bags. Either way, they just need preparing with hot water for a very beneficial drink.

Tinctures

A tincture usually contains alcohol which is used to extract and concentrate the active properties of the herb. Tinctures are very easily assimilated by the body and are therefore a very easy and effective way to take a herbal product. If you wish to lessen the effect of the alcohol, then pour the tincture into a small amount of very hot water for a few minutes. The alcohol will vaporize and after it has cooled, it will be ready to drink.

Herbal products, unlike drugs, will take time to provide a beneficial effect in the body. The time scale could be a few weeks to a few months, depending on what the herbal preparation is being used for.

The reason for this is that the herb will supply various "actions" in the body. First a cleansing or neutralizing action; next possibly an antiseptic action, followed by a deodorizing action, and finally a building action to re-build the body back to full health. As you can appreciate, all this takes time, but it is well worth the wait in the long run.

The quality of the raw material used will determine the potency of the finished herbal product. Therefore it is well worth while doing a little research on a particular supplier or manufacturer before you part with your money.

Do You Live In a European Union Country?

Of particular concern in Europe. In 2011 the European Union introduced the Herbal Medicines Directive which means the herbal industry has been all but destroyed by a draconian law which has virtually banned the supply of herbal products within the European Union.

The excuse for issuing this directive is "to ensure public safety with regard to herbal products". I would have thought that something that has been used safely for hundreds (and in some cases thousands) of years would be safe for the public to take.

Many herbal products have been classified, not for use in food preparation (i.e. for cooking or garnishing purposes) but as "medicines" and a company now needs a license in order to sell them to the public. The cost of the license is in the order of $150,000 per herbal product. Yes, you read that correctly, $150,000 per herbal product.

Say you are a manufacturer and have just a small range of just 20 herbal products, that is going to cost you $3,000,000 in license fees, before you can sell anything. Very few manufacturers have that kind of money to waste on licenses for something that has been used safely for all those years.

All this new law is going to do is drive the supply of these safe, natural herbal products underground. With the power of modern communications and the Internet, all you have to do is spend a little time seeking out those herbal products you require from sources outside Europe. Many suppliers in other parts of the world—and especially the United States—will be more than happy to supply you, and will ship their products internationally. As the saying goes—where there's a will there's a way!!

When buying any herbal product, make sure there are no artificial fillers, binders or artificial sugar coatings. Tablets can contain magnesium stearate or stearic acid which is used as a lubricant in the manufacturing process. Binders can be added to help hold the ingredients together. Often artificial colors are added to make the product look good. A shellac coating can be added which will be listed in the ingredients as "natural glaze." Capsules can have fillers added to fill-up the capsule.

Only buy natural herbal products—not synthetic ones. Make sure you do your research on the supplier / manufacturer before purchasing.

An A to Z of Herbs

Alfalfa

Alfalfa is a grass which contains all the essential amino acids as well as being rich in trace minerals and enzymes. It is frequently taken to lessen the effects of hay fever allergies. It is also fed to horses as a counter to arthritic conditions and digestive problems.

As it is a good source of fiber, it is useful for detoxifying the body in addition to improving liver health.

Barberry

Barberry has been valued for its antibiotic action for over 2,000 years. The active ingredient in Barberry—Berberine is a very potent fighter against bacterial infections. In addition it also stimulates the immune system and assists in reducing high blood pressure due to its ability to dilate blood vessels.

It has a very positive action on the liver—assisting in the flow of bile which is important in all liver conditions, but especially jaundice.

Basil

Basil is often thought of as a culinary product—especially for use in pasta sauce. However, it has been used for thousands of years to treat a variety of ailments including intestinal parasites and worms as well as being an excellent treatment for other intestinal conditions.

Indian researchers have also used Basil Oil successfully to treat various skin infections such as acne.

Basil is also useful in drawing out poisons from wasp and hornet stings as well as the venom from snake bites.

As it is an excellent antispasmodic, it is also helpful in cases of whooping cough

Bayberry

Used by early American settlers for a variety of conditions including: colds and flu when combined with ginger or capsicum. The root bark contains an antibiotic chemical called myricitrin which has the ability to combat various bacteria strains as well as protozoa.

Myricitrin also play a key role in alleviating the effects of diarrhea and dysentery, in addition to reducing the effects of fever.

Bayberry also supports the adrenal glands as well as being a blood cleanser and removing waste material from arteries and veins.

Bilberry

Bilberry and its close cousin blueberry are often confused as they each have a dark blue smooth skin. Bilberry has been used for medicinal purposes in Europe since the 16th century. By comparison, blueberry has been widely cultivated in the US since the 1920s. They are both potent antioxidants and are therefore excellent free radial scavengers.

Bilberry (and blueberry) is often associated with providing benefits for eye vision. This was apparent during World War 11 when bomber pilots flying night bombing missions over occupied Europe found that their night vision improved if they ate bilberry jam before leaving on their missions.

Bilberry strengthens the tiny capillaries that surround the eyes. In so doing, it improves circulation and thus increases the ability of fluids and nutrients to more easily pass through.

However, eye vision is not the only benefits derived from bilberry. Bilberry is excellent for supporting the entire circulatory system. It improves circulation to the hands, feet, brain and heart. The incidence of blood clots can be reduced as well as reducing the risk of atherosclerosis.

By combining bilberry with vitamin E, the formation of cataracts can be reduced; it also has the ability to protect the eyes from the effects of diabetes.

Blackberry

Blackberry is often associated with jam or is often eaten as berries. However, it has tremendous medicinal properties.

Because it has an high tannin content—which makes it more astringent—this makes it an excellent treatment for diarrhea and dysentery. This astringent action also makes it useful in wound healing as it constricts blood vessels and stops minor bleeding.

Eating the berries can help alleviate the effects of mouth sores as well as the effects of a sore throat. And finally, it has uses as a treatment for hemorrhoids due to its astringent action.

Black Cohosh

Black Cohosh is widely used to treat menopausal symptoms such as hot flashes, night sweats, migraines, mood swings, heart palpitations and dryness. The roots of the plant are used medically and are available as capsules, a liquid extract or tablets.

Black Walnut

Traditionally used as a nutritional aid for the intestinal system, Black Walnut has the same laxative action as cascara sagrada, but it works more gently. Due to its astringent qualities, black walnut has the power to assist the body in protecting itself from harmful agents such as parasitic worms. It also has an high iodine content, which is good for energy as it supports thyroid function.

Blessed Thistle

Blessed Thistle has many uses in the herbal medicine chest. It is a memory booster by supplying oxygen to the brain. It helps reduce fevers. It is a great herb for females in assisting with the effects of menopausal problems. Blessed Thistle also supports the digestive system and is an overall tonic for the body.

Blue Cohosh

Blue Cohosh is not related to Black Cohosh—they originate in different botanical families. Native Americans called Blue Cohosh papoose root thinking that it triggered labor and hastened childbirth.

In addition to its use to induce labor, it has historically also been used to treat cases of arthritis, epilepsy, hiccups, infant colic and sore throat.

As it is an antispasmodic, Blue Cohosh also supports the nervous system. It is especially useful for relieving muscle cramps and spasms.

Blue Vervain

Blue Vervain is one of the best herbs to take to alleviate the effects of the common cold. For bronchial problems Blue Vervain has the ability to remove phlegm from the chest.

Blue Vervain also supports the nervous system and in this role it acts as a natural tranquilizer and creates a calming and relaxing feeling.

Boneset

Boneset has nothing to do with repairing broken bones!

This herb is an effective treatment for bacterial and viral infections. It achieves this by stimulating the immune system to attack these foreign invaders.

Native Americans introduced Boneset to early colonists as a sweat-inducer to relieve the effects of a fever, such as: influenza, cholera, dengue fever, malaria and typhoid. It was also used to treat an arthritic condition as well as treating appetite loss, constipation and indigestion.

Buckthorn

Buckthorn is a very potent laxative which was widely used in Europe during the 13th century. In more recent times it has been used for other purposes such as: arthritis, gout, hemorrhoids, jaundice and to promote menstruation. When taken hot it induces sweating which will reduce a fever. When used as an ointment, the herb will reduce itching. If the leaves are bruised and applied to a wound it will stop small amounts of bleeding.

Burdock

Burdock Root is one of the best blood purifiers to clear circulatory and lymphatic congestion. As it assists in alleviating excess body fluids, toxins are more easily purged from the body.

Other uses for burdock root: aids in reducing swelling around joints, expels surplus calcium deposits and cleanses the blood of harmful acids.

Butchers Broom

Butchers Broom has been used for hundreds of years to provide support to the circulatory system—and with circulatory system conditions being the number one killer in the United States—this herb could prove very beneficial for many Americans.

Butchers Broom strengthens blood vessel walls, making it ideal in cases of post-operative surgery to prevent thrombosis. It is also used to treat hemorrhoids, phlebitis and varicose veins.

It increases blood circulation to the brain which can aid in memory function. Additionally, it can help prevent heart problems by reducing cholesterol levels and helping prevent atherosclerosis—a disease where plaque builds up inside arteries.

Capsicum

Capsicum also called cayenne has a warming effect and is often used to treat instances of cold hands and cold feet. As such it is an excellent circulatory product. It has also gained a good reputation as a painkiller and digestive aid. The main active ingredient is capsaicin—an oily phytochemical. Additionally, it has been used to relieve symptoms of a cold and sore throat.

Caraway

Caraway seed is something that is often thought of as an addition to rye bread. Why is it added to rye bread and other foods? The reason: since ancient times it has been used to support the digestive tract and expel gas.

In modern times, researchers have discovered that two oils in caraway seed—carvol and carvene—soothe the smooth muscle of the digestive tract, and it is these oils that make caraway so effective. Caraway is not only used to support the digestive system, but it also has an antispasmodic action which is a useful treatment for women who experience menstrual cramps.

Cascara Sagrada

Well known for its quick acting laxative effects. It is often used for constipation in addition to helping purge toxins from the body. It promotes peristaltic action—the movement of waste matter through the colon, and stimulates secretions from the gall bladder, liver, pancreas and stomach.

Catnip

A member of the mint family, Catnip has been used for thousands of years from Europe to China. One of its main uses is to sooth the digestive tract, but also to alleviate the effects of a cold. Native Americans used it for infant colic; and as it has a mild tranquilizer action, it has also been used to promote restful sleep, as well as provide support for the nervous system.

As Catnip is a spasmodic, it is often used to relieve menstrual cramps.

Catnip also possesses antibiotic properties which make it useful for treating diarrhea and to reduce the effects of a fever.

Celery

We often think of celery as something to add to salads to chew on—but researchers have found quite a few benefits in celery seeds. These benefits include: providing relief from anxiety and insomnia—celery contains natural chemicals which have a sedative effect. Chinese researchers have successfully used celery with people who suffer from high blood pressure. Various studies have shown that celery seed can reduce blood sugar (glucose) levels, which is an important component of managing diabetes.

Celery contains a natural diuretic which can help with weight loss—especially if someone is obese as it will tend to eliminate water weight. However, it is important to bear in mind that any water weight lost will tend to return. The only real answer to sustained—and maintained weight loss is to change the diet into one that is low in saturated fat and high in fiber and complex carbohydrates, coupled with an appropriate exercise program.

Chamomile

Dried chamomile flowers were used in ancient Egypt, Greece and Rome to treat many disorders of the body, including anxiety, stress and sleeping problems. This was achieved by its calming and sedative effect. In more recent times it has been used as a tea for relaxation and as a sleep aid.

Chaparral

Chaparral has very strong antioxidant properties in addition to it being an antiseptic, pain killer and having anti-tumor actions.

In its antiseptic form, it is often used as a mouthwash to fight tooth decay, and pyorrhea—inflammation of the gums. One study shows that a Chaparral mouthwash reduced cavities by 75 percent.

As a tumor fighter, the National Cancer Institute has received numerous testimonials from different individuals claiming that it cured their cancers. In fact several studies have shown that it does shrink cancer tumors.

Chickweed

Chickweed is used to strengthen the colon and stomach as well as helping to dissolve plaque and fatty deposits. Chickweed has healing properties for stomach ulcers and inflammation in the colon.

Cloves

Cloves are a good natural parasite cleansing herb which can be obtained as a liquid, powder or in a capsule.

Coltsfoot

Coltsfoot is best known as a cough suppressant and to support the respiratory system. This herb has a high mucilage and saponin content which acts as a disinfectant and anti-inflammatory agent for respiratory problems.

The flowers have expectorant properties which mean they are very soothing to mucus membranes and are especially beneficial for chest and lung conditions.

Comfrey

Comfrey contains a chemical called Allantoin which helps with the growth of new cells. This chemical is the reason why comfrey is well known as a wound healer and to knit broken bones together. Comfrey has been used for centuries for these two purposes.

As comfrey secretes its natural hormone to the pituitary gland, it helps to strengthen the structural system.

Comfrey also supports the digestive system by helping the secretion of pepsin and it is a general aid for the respiratory system. In fact, comfrey is a general aid and tonic for the whole body.

Cranberry

Cranberry's main purpose is to treat bacterial infections in the bladder. It is often combined with buchu herb.

When used together, these two herbs have anti-inflammatory, diuretic and antiseptic properties. Scientific studies show that cranberry makes the urinary tract inhospitable to bacteria, thus lessening the risk of urinary tract infections. Buchu acts as a diuretic and improves digestion. This product works best in acidic urine conditions.

Damiana

Damiana is one of the most popular herbal products to restore normal sexual function in males by increasing sperm count, and for strengthening the egg in females. In addition, it helps to balance female hormones. It is helpful in increasing sexual strength in those who have a weak libido.

Dandelion

Dandelion has been used for centuries to stimulate the liver to detoxify poisons. It is important for promoting good circulatory system function and strengthening weak arteries.

Dong Quai

Dong Quai—a member of the celery family—is one of the oldest known herbs, having been used in China, Japan and Korea for over 1,000 years. It is primarily known as a women's product, to relieve menopausal symptoms such as: hot flashes, menstrual disorders such as cramps, irregular menstrual cycles, infrequent periods, premenstrual syndrome (PMS), and menopausal symptoms.

It is suggested that Dong Quai contains compounds that may help reduce pain, dilate blood vessels, and stimulate and relax uterine muscles.

In traditional Chinese medicine (TCM), different parts of the dong quai root are used for different actions in the body: the root head is used as an anticoagulant, the main part of the root is used as a tonic, and the tail-end of the root is used to remove blood stagnation. Because it is a balancer of the female hormonal system, it is often called "female's ginseng."

Echinacea

There are various strains of Echinacea. It is used to support the immune system and is involved in the production of white blood cells, which assists the body to fight infection. Echinacea purges toxins from the blood and enhances lymphatic drainage.

Echinacea contains polysaccharides that stimulate the production of phagocytes (cells that engulf and consume foreign matter) and activate T -lymphocytes, macrophages and natural killer cells. Taken at the earliest sign of a cold or infection, echinacea may help cut recovery time considerably.

Elderberry

One of the oldest known herbs. It works in the respiratory and immune body systems, and is usually used to counter the effects of colds, flu, congestion, sore throat and inflammation.

Elecampane

Used for over 1,000 years, elecampane is probably best known for expelling intestinal parasites and worms. But that is not all; it is also effective as a respiratory system support—especially for the elimination of catarrh. As it is one of the richest natural sources of insulin it is highly beneficial for the pancreas.

Eucalyptus

Have you ever used Listerine mouthwash or Vicks VapaRub, if so then you have come into contact with Eucalyptus? Eucalyptus Oil is very potent and is therefore excellent for loosening phlegm in the chest, making it easier for it to be expelled. It is also used to treat cases of pyorrhea—inflammation of the gums.

Eucalyptus provides an anti-bacterial action against infections in minor cuts and wounds. Studies in Russia have determined that Eucalyptus kills the influenza virus—a virus that causes flu.

Fennel Seed

Fennel Seed has several uses including: supporting the digestive and nervous systems, alleviating the effects of colic, gas and intestinal problems. It also has diuretic properties.

Fenugreek

Fenugreek comprises various components including saponins, alkaloids and fiber. It is a respiratory system herb which assists in expelling mucous, phlegm and infections from the lungs, and toxic waste through the lymphatic system. In addition, Fenugreek is able to dissolve a hardened build up of mucous which can then be eliminated.

Garcinia Cambogia

Garcinia Cambogia is a tropical fruit which contains HCA (hydroxy-citric acid), which stimulates the body to burn carbohydrates as energy rather than storing them as fat. HCA acts as an appetite suppressant which gives a feeling of fullness, thus reducing the intake of food, therefore reducing fat and cholesterol formation.

Garlic

This popular herb offers a boost to the immune system with its antibacterial, antifungal and antiviral properties. It is excellent for purging candida yeast and parasites from the body.

Garlic has so many uses from using it in cooking to it being an excellent product for heart health. Other recognized health benefits of garlic include: acting as an antibiotic and having anti-cholesterol and anti-hypertensive properties.

It is also an antioxidant which protects the body against the effects of free radical damage. Its high sulphur content assists in cell purification.

Allicin is the principle biological active compound which gives garlic its odor. Be warned. Many so called "odorless" garlic products have the active compound removed which makes it rather worthless. It can be obtained as a garlic bulb, in a capsule or in tablet form.

Garlic has many uses:

- Anti-biotic - natural penicillin
- Arteriosclerosis
- Arthritis
- Asthma

- Blood poisoning
- High blood pressure
- Anti-viral
- Anti-bacterial
- Destroys many types of parasites
- For respiratory conditions use with mullein or lobelia
- As a decongestant / expectorant use with lobelia
- For bacterial infection use with golden seal, echinacea, pau d'arco
- For viral infection use with colloidal silver
- For yeast infections use with pau d'arco
- For swollen lymph nodes use with lobelia and mullein
- For parasites use with pumpkin seeds and black walnut

Gentian

Gentian Root helps in the breakdown of fats and proteins and assists in the body's assimilation of iron and vitamin B12. As it has a cooling effect on body tissue, this helps reduce infections and inflammation. Gentian Root also promotes digestive secretions.

Ginger

Ginger Root is an excellent cleansing agent for the colon, skin and kidneys. It provides support to the respiratory system. It is often used to alleviate the effects of a cold or flu. Many people take it as a natural alternative for motion and morning sickness.

Ginkgo Biloba

Ginkgo Biloba, an antioxidant herb, promotes increased circulation. It also dilates blood vessels and bronchioles to improve circulation and oxygenation of cells. It also has scientifically proven nervous-system benefits in addition to improving memory function.

Golden Seal

Golden Seal has infection-fighting abilities and anti-inflammatory properties. It can be used as an alternative to cranberry if required.

Gotu Kola

Gotu Kola originates from Sri Lanka. It is used extensively in Ayurvedic medicine where its prime purpose is to support the nervous system and especially the brain. It is therefore often referred to as "food for the brain". It is a nervous system tonic where it generates energy within the cells of the brain, and as a result, it escalates physical and mental power as well as stimulating the pituitary gland.

It is used to treat nervous system disorders including epilepsy, memory loss and schizophrenia, and is also used to treat the effects of aging.

Gotu Kola's primary use for centuries was to treat serious skin conditions such as bruises, elephantitis and leprosy (which is now called Hansen's disease), psoriasis and syphilitic ulcers.

A study published in the British journal *Nature* supported the use of Gotu Kola for the treatment of leprosy. The bacteria that causes leprosy has a waxy coating which protects them from white blood cells in the immune system designed to destroy them. Gotu Kola contains a chemical (asiaticoside) which destroys this wax coating which enables the bacteria to be eliminated.

A cream containing Gotu Kola applied to painful scaly psoriasis welts can bring relief. Various studies have shown that Gotu Kola improves circulation in the lower limbs. Further studies are underway to determine if Gotu Kola would be suitable for treating varicose veins.

Grapefruit Seed Extract

Grapefruit Seed Extract is an effective anti-parasitic herb which has a very bitter taste. This can be sweetened by adding a small amount of honey.

Gymnema Sylvestre

Gymnema Sylvestre is a climbing plant which is native to Australia, parts of Africa and central and southern India, and is used in Ayurvedic medicine. It is primarily used for weight management to control appetite and cravings, but has also been used to treat constipation and diabetes

Hawthorn Berries

Hawthorn is known as the heart herb. It improves circulation and heart strength. In studies, hawthorn recipients also reported fewer overall heart symptoms, less fatigue and less shortness of breath.

It is often taken along with ginkgo biloba to improve circulation especially to the heart.

Hibiscus Flower

Hibiscus Flower has anti-bacterial properties as well as being an anti-parasitic. In addition, it acts as a diuretic and has a soothing effect.

Hops

Hops have three primary medicinal functions: as a sedative, digestive aid and for women health. Of the three, it is best known for its sedative qualities on the nervous system, and for inducing sleep in cases of insomnia.

According to French researchers, hops has antispasmodic properties which improves digestion by relaxing the muscle lining of the digestive tract.

German researchers state that hops contains alkaloids similar to the female sex hormone estrogen which promotes menstruation.

Horehound

Horehound has been used for over 2000 years as an herbal expectorant and cough remedy. Horehound contains an alkaloid (marrubiin) which loosens phlegm. Horehound also has the ability to stimulate bile secretions and is also used for wound healing.

Horehound acts as a tonic to the respiratory system as well as the stomach. It has also been used successfully when applied topically for such skin conditions as the herpes simplex virus, eczema and shingles.

Horsetail

This herb has diuretic properties and can help with some kidney conditions. It is particularly effective as a healing agent when blood is present in the urine. Horsetail also has astringent properties and as such, is used for bed-wetting in children and incontinence in adults.

Horsetail is rich in silica, which helps to soothe and strengthen connective tissue. Silica is required for bone and cartilage formation, as well as assisting the body in absorbing and utilizing calcium. Calcium is needed for repairing fractures and treating bone diseases, including rickets and osteoporosis. Horsetail is used to strengthen bones, teeth, nails and hair. The improvements in cartilage formation helps to lessen inflammation and combat joint pain, arthritis, gout, muscle cramps, hemorrhoids, spasms and rheumatism.

The silica content in Horsetail also promotes the growth of collagen—a protein which is found in connective tissue. Collagen assists in improving skin health and tone.

Hydrangea

Hydrangea is best known as a treatment for kidney and bladder stones. Kidney stones are made of mineral and acid salts which form into hard deposits inside the kidneys. Many things can cause kidney stones to form, but one of the most common causes is not drinking enough fluids during the day—ideally filtered water.

Most often kidney stones form when the urine becomes concentrated and this allows minerals to crystalize and clump together. Hydrangea helps stop these deposits from forming—which cause severe pain when they pass from the kidneys through the ureters to the bladder.

Recent studies show that Hydrangea can reduce inflammation of the prostate gland and improve prostate health. Adding Horsetail can increase the effectiveness of the treatment.

Herbalists recommend Hydrangea for many conditions of the urinary system including: cystitis, benign prostatic hyperplasia (BPH), dysuria, edema, incontinence, inflammation and tumor formation.

Hyssop

You can find Hyssop mentioned in the Bible. In the Book of Psalms (51:9) *"Purge me with Hyssop and I shall be clean"*. There is more to "cleaning" than mentioned in the Bible. In fact Hyssop is often used to induce sweating to reduce fevers; and leaves can be applied to wounds to help reduce infections and assist in the healing process.

Hyssop has been used successfully as a gargle to treat nose and throat infections, and used as an infusion for a cough, where phlegm and congestion are involved, which develops from having a cold. Camphor-like compounds in Hyssop help to expectorate phlegm. It is also an aid for poor digestion as well as to treat breast and lung problems. It has also been used to expel mucus in the intestines.

Used as an infusion in a compress Hyssop restricts the growth of the Herpes Simplex virus which causes cold sores, as well as the Genital Herpes virus.

Juniper

Juniper is used for several conditions in herbal healing. In the urinary system, because Juniper contains a chemical terpinene-4-0l which has diuretic properties, it is often used where uric acid is being retained in addition to excess water retention; it is also used to treat cases of high blood pressure.

Diuretics assist in relieving the bloated feeling caused by premenstrual fluid retention. Females concerned with premenstrual syndrome may obtain benefits by trying Juniper during the stressful days prior to their monthly periods.

Juniper has been found to be especially useful for treating prostate and urinary tract infections in men who suffer from benign prostatic hypertrophy (BPH). It is also a useful herb for treating cases of bacteria and yeast infections.

A liquid extract can be made from Juniper Berries and used as a gargle for mouth and throat infections.

Juniper also has anti-inflammatory properties which makes it a useful herb for arthritic conditions.

Because of its high chromium content, Juniper has also been used to treat blood sugar imbalances.

Kava Kava

Kava Kava is very effective at treating anxiety and depression. It has a natural sedative effect which does not affect alertness unlike some medications. It should not be taken for more than six months at a time unless advised otherwise by a qualified practitioner.

Kelp

Kelp is a sea vegetable which is harvested at low tide. It is an excellent source of iodine and in 1750 a British physician introduced a cure for goiter—a thyroid enlargement caused by thyroid deficiency—by mixing vegetable oil with charred kelp. In fact no one knew how his concoction worked until 1812 when scientists realized there was iodine in the kelp plant and that goiters were caused by iodine deficiency.

In fact Kelp provides good support for the glandular system, as it assists with control of the thyroid gland and helps regulate the metabolism which is involved with food digestion.

Kelp has also been used in cases of obesity due to its iodine content and its function within the thyroid gland.

In addition to iodine, Kelp also contains sodium alginate which is beneficial for health problems associated with heavy metal toxicity, radiation and heart disease.

In addition to the above, kelp also has many uses including: anemia, arthritis, asthma, candida yeast infections, coughs, diabetes, prostate and ovarian problems, fatigue, fungal infections, high blood pressure, ulcers and skin conditions such as eczema and psoriasis.

Kelp is a rich source of nutrients including almost every mineral and trace mineral required by the human body.

Korean Ginseng

Korean Ginseng—also called Panax Ginseng—has been used for over 5,000 years as a preventative tonic to nourish the whole body, especially for stress, fatigue and weak conditions. It grows primarily in China, South Korea and Japan.

Korean Ginseng is considered the strongest form of ginseng. Ginsenoside compounds found in Korean Ginseng assist in lowering blood sugar levels, while polysaccharides help to enhance the immune system. Antioxidant properties help to stimulate the immune system to help protect the body from various diseases and stress.

Korean Ginseng assists in the production of endorphins which makes a person feel exhilarated. It also has significant sexual health benefits to help improve erectile function, and increase testosterone levels and sperm count.

Kudzu

Historically Asian-Healers have used Kudzu to treat colds, flu, high blood pressure, allergies and many other ailments.

More recently, Chinese-Healers have used Kudzu to treat people who have an alcohol dependency. It has also been used with St John's Wort to treat the depressive effects of alcohol withdrawal. Kudzu is available in capsules, tablets, and as a dried root.

Lavender

Lavender can be used in different ways to treat anxiety, tension, headaches and insomnia. It is usually steeped in hot water so that the steam can be inhaled. Other options are to make it into a tea or it can be used as an essential oil and massaged into the skin. This will help manage stress and improve mood, concentration and reduce anxiety. Lavender has the ability to relax the nervous system and improve sleep patterns.

Lemon Balm

Lemon Balm is a calmative for the nerves and as a result, relieves tension in the body. Its effect is soothing and it is used for treating anxiety and stress.

Licorice

Licorice has long been recognized for the natural sweetness of its deep-sinking roots. Next to ginseng, licorice is the most popular herb used in Chinese formulas. It helps support the adrenal glands during periods of stress.

Lobelia

Lobelia has a lengthy history of use as an herbal remedy for respiratory conditions such as asthma, bronchitis, pneumonia, and cough. Traditionally, Native Americans smoked lobelia as a treatment for asthma. Today, some herbalists use lobelia to help clear mucus from the respiratory tract, including the throat, lungs, and bronchial tubes. Additionally, Lobelia is used as part of a comprehensive treatment plan for asthma.

Maca

Maca, also known as Peruvian Ginseng is used to increase stamina, energy and sexual function in both men and women. In one study, researchers found that Maca may help alleviate sexual dysfunction caused by the use of selective-serotonin re-uptake inhibitors (SSRIs) which are used in the treatment of depression.

Marjoram

Marjoram is often taken for motion sickness as well as to soothe the digestive tract where it acts as an antispasmodic. For women it is often used in cases of menstrual cramps.

Marjoram can inhibit the growth of the herpes simplex virus which is responsible for cold sores and genital herpes. Due to its calmative and stimulant properties, it is often used in cases of asthma, coughs and other respiratory disorders..

Marshmallow

This mucilant soothes the kidneys when they are irritated or inflamed. Marshmallow contains volatile oils and tannins that are responsible for its diuretic actions. It is especially helpful in passing kidney stones.

Milk Thistle

This natural support to the liver contains a mixture of bioflavonoids, including silymarin. Milk Thistle strengthens the liver against auto-intoxication and stimulates protein synthesis in liver cells, which generates DNA and RNA.

Mullein

Mullein has both mucilant and astringent properties. Its powerful healing abilities make it useful for healing weak lung tissue and chronic respiratory congestion. It has a proven expectorant action that likely arises from saponin compounds in the plant. Scientific studies suggest that the mucilage in mullein protects mucous membranes, preventing cell invasion by viral allergens.

Myrrh

Myrrh originates in the Middle East where it has been used for thousands of years. It is mentioned several times in the Bible. Probably the best known reference concerns Joseph and how his jealous brothers plotted to get rid of this pesky sibling—without actually killing him—whose father thought he could do no wrong.

One day the answer to their problem presented itself "*And looking up, they saw a caravan of Ishmaelites coming from Gilead, with their camels bearing gum, balm and myrrh on their way to carry it down to Egypt*" (Genesis 37:25). So they sold Joseph to the Ishmaelites. You can read the rest of the story in the Bible!

Today Myrrh is used for oral hygiene. As a mouthwash, it contains tannins which have an astringent action on tissue. It also has an anti-inflammatory action in addition to fighting bacteria.

It is also used to treat mouth ulcers and bleeding gums. In addition, herbalists recommend adding powered myrrh to wounds that have been well cleansed to act as an antiseptic. It can also be mixed with water to use as a gargle to treat a sore throat. It can also be used to treat colds, coughs asthma and congestion of the chest.

Myrrh provides support and strength to the digestive system as well as assisting with waste elimination.

Myrrh is often added to "natural" toothpaste—the best place to look for it is in health food stores—where it is used to help fight the bacteria which cause tooth decay.

Nettle

We often think of nettle as a nuisance weed that stings—and therefore has to be destroyed at all cost! However, it has many uses in herbal medicine. In Germany it is prescribed for circulatory system support and to reduce high blood pressure. Because of its high vitamin C content it is traditionally used to prevent scurvy.

As the plant contains alkaloids which neutralize uric acid, it is used to treat cases of rheumatism. Native American women drank nettle tea during pregnancy to strengthen the fetus and ease delivery. It was also used by them to stop cases of uterine bleeding after childbirth.

The root of the plant contains tannins which have been used as an enema to shrink hemorrhoids. Nettle can also be used as a tonic to strengthen the whole body.

Nettle is highly nutritious. You can boil or steam the young leaves and eat them as a vegetable. When the stems are boiled, they lose their sting. They can therefore be used in salads.

Nopal

Nopal or Mexican Cactus as it is sometimes called is traditionally used by the Mexicans as a food especially in salads. The nutritional factors in nopal act in the bowel to prevent fat and excessive sugars from entering the bloodstream. By helping the body maintain balanced blood sugar levels, Nopal aids the body in its battle against obesity. Additionally, it is used as an anti-inflammatory, as a laxative and as a hypoglycemic vehicle for diabetes and gastritis.

Oatstraw

Oatstraw is a good source of minerals for nourishing bones, hair, skin and nails. It helps calm the nervous system and can assist in cases of depression and nervous exhaustion.

Olive Leaf Extract

Olive Leaf Extract supports normal blood pressure and cholesterol levels and strengthens the immune system against viral and bacterial attacks.

Oregon Grape

Oregon Grape is mainly used as a blood cleanser where there are toxins in the blood which cause skin diseases such as eczema, psoriasis, herpes and acne. It also supports thyroid function, and is in fact a tonic for all the glandular system.

It supports a healthy liver and gall bladder by increasing bile flow, and as it has antibacterial properties it is often used to treat a candida yeast overgrowth, diarrhea, parasites and urinary tract infections.

Oregano

Available in either enteric coated (meaning it will burst in the body where it is supposed to), or in liquid form. Oregano possesses anti-inflammatory antiviral and anti-fungal properties which makes it especially useful for eradicating candida yeast.

Parsley

Parsley is probably one of the best known herbs as it is used in culinary dishes as well as for medicinal uses. It comes in a variety of different "leaf types", from feather like to curled to flat. The flat leafed variety is most often used for medicinal purposes.

It is used to treat urinary tract infections, indigestion, to relieve the effects of gas and as a digestive aid. Additionally, it is a natural body deodorizer and eradicates bad breath.

Passion Flower

A natural sedative, passionflower will help you sleep without leaving a groggy feeling the next morning. It is beneficial for calming the nervous system, and for when the body is under stress.

Passion Flower slows the breakdown of neurotransmitters which pass chemical messages between the body's cells, as well as working with certain enzymes. It also assists in calming an irritable bowel, as well as killing certain bacteria.

Pau D'Arco

Pau D'Arco is native to South America. It contains a chemical called lapachol, which may provide nutritional support to the immune system. It is commonly used against many conditions of unwanted growth, including fungus, yeast and tumors as well as fungal infections. Historically, it has also been used to remedy the side effects of some antibiotics.

It is available as a capsule, tablet or as a lotion.

Pennyroyal

A member of the mint family, Pennyroyal contains a chemical (pulegone) within its oil that is often used as an insect repellent— especially against mosquitoes, fleas, gnats, flies and ticks. In fact several natural insect killers contain the oil from Pennyroyal.

Pennyroyal is also used as a decongestant and cough remedy due to its strong aromatic smell, which acts as a decongestant. It also supports the digestive system in cases of stomach discomfort and bloating where it will expel gas.

Peppermint

Peppermint stimulates the production of digestive fluids. It also eradicates bad breath and helps settle an upset stomach. If purchased in liquid form, then only tiny drops should be applied to water, otherwise it will be too strong.

Psyllium

Psyllium is an excellent source of fiber—and is especially useful for those individuals who suffer from celiac disease as it contains no gluten. It is important to drink plenty of water with Psyllium as this helps it work better.

Psyllium acts as a sponge in the colon, soaking up toxins which can then be eliminated. It is non-irritating to the mucus membranes in the intestinal tract, but instead, strengthens and tones them.

Pumpkin Seeds

One of the best tasting of all the anti-parasite herbal products. The seeds can be eaten as a snack. In fact they taste so good that you cannot eat enough of them. Pumpkin Seeds are very effective against tapeworms as well as other types of parasites. They also serve as a good source of essential fatty acids (EFAs) which are essential for good health.

Pygeum Extract

Obtained from the bark of a tree in Africa, Pygeum is used to prevent and relieve benign prostate enlargement, it contains anti-inflammatory phytosterol compounds in addition to triterpenoid compounds which have an anti-swelling effect.

Red Clover

Red Clover has been cultivated as forage since prehistoric times. In more recent times, red clover has been used as a cancer treatment for non-estrogen dependent cancers. Researchers from the National Cancer Institute (NCI) have identified four anti tumor compounds in red clover. They also discovered that a high concentration of tocopherol—a form of the antioxidant vitamin E was also present in the plant.

In addition, studies show that red clover acts like the female sex hormone estrogen, which means it may alleviate menopausal symptoms. Red Clover also supports the nervous system in cases of nervous exhaustion.

Red Raspberry

This herb is renowned for its nutritional support of the female reproductive system. Red Raspberry is known to nourish and strengthen the uterus. A common backyard fruit bush, red raspberry is an excellent herbal source of iron, manganese and niacin. It also contains quantities of vitamins C, A, D, E and B, as well as phosphorus and calcium.

Rosemary

Rosemary, a member of the mint family is an excellent tonic and improves circulation and supports the nervous system as well as enhancing the memory. It complements other members of the mint family in addition to lavender and other herbs. It can be used in various forms. For example:

Rosemary Leaf Extract

Rosemary Leaf Extract as well as being excellent for the nervous system, it also supports the digestive system where problems arise due to emotional stress. In addition, it is also an excellent antibacterial and has astringent properties.

Rosemary Tea

Rosemary Tea has been drunk for centuries to ease the effects of headaches as well as improving circulation and neutralizing some of the effects of memory loss. It can help when working long hours or studying to help keep the mind focused on the task at hand. Like rosemary leaf extract, it is also beneficial for the digestive system. Cold rosemary tea can be used as an antibacterial mouth wash.

Saffron

Spain is the world's leading exporter of Saffron which was introduced into the country in the 8th century by the Arabs. It helps protect against heart disease by reducing cholesterol through deactivating uric acid build-up. In parts of Spain where Saffron is grown and eaten on a daily basis, there are very few instances of heart disease.

In Indian Ayurvedic medicine Saffron is used to stimulate the circulatory system, and is used for kidney and liver conditions.

Sage

This aromatic herb is probably best known at Thanksgiving for being used in turkey stuffing. However, culinary uses aside; it is also an important herb in the herbal medicine chest.

It has been used historically as an antiperspirant and to reduce fevers. Scientific studies have determined that Sage will cut perspiration by up to 50 per cent approximately two hours after ingestion. This is why it proved so useful to reduce sweating from fever.

Sage has been used as a treatment for wound healing due to its anti-bacterial activity. It is also a potent antioxidant and as such, it has been used to preserve meat. In fact, it is often used to inhibit bacteria growth in hamburger meat prior to the meat being grilled on a barbecue. Food hygiene is an important consideration especially when meat may be left out for extended periods of time in a warm sunny environment. Bacteria in meat can cause stomach upsets as well as food poisoning.

Sage steeped in warm water can be used as a gargle for sore throat and tonsillitis. A study conducted in Germany determined that Sage made into an infusion and consumed on an empty stomach can reduce blood sugar levels in diabetics.

Sarsaparilla

Historically Sarsaparilla was used as a blood purifier to treat syphilis—which was quite common in 19th century America. In more recent times it has been used to treat colds, cough, fever and gout.

Sarsaparilla supports the glandular system and contains the male hormone testosterone, as well as progesterone—a female hormone produced in the ovaries.

Saw Palmetto

Saw Palmetto is mainly used to treat benign prostatic hyperplasia (BPH). BPH is a male condition which includes frequent urination, difficulty in fulfilling the urge to urinate, dribbling after urination, a weak urinary stream, and finally, waking up several times at night to urinate.

Shepherds Purse

Shepherds Purse contains compounds that assist in blood clotting—and therefore this herb is useful to stop bleeding from wounds. It is also used to treat hemorrhoids due to its astringent action.

It is also used to constrict blood vessels and is therefore useful to control either high or low blood pressure as well as heart function.

Siberian Ginseng

Siberian Ginseng (Eleuthero) contains compounds called ginsenosides which alleviate stress and boost mental and physical performance. It has been used for centuries in Russia and China as an adaptogen—meaning, it allows the body to relax during stressful periods. It also helps balance neurotransmitters such as serotonin and dopamine in the brain. In addition to helping balance blood sugar levels, it also enhances a sense of well-being.

Skullcap

Skullcap is a member of the mint family and is traditionally used as a nerve tonic as well as a sedative for relieving anxiety and insomnia. In addition it relieves nervous exhaustion and supports the nervous system.

Slippery Elm

Slippery elm is very soothing to inflamed tissue—especially in the gastrointestinal tract—and as a result, is excellent for tissue healing. It is easily digested and offers good laxative properties.

St. John's Wort

This popular herb has gained national attention for its ability to alleviate mild to moderate depression. It contains an active constituent, hypericin, which appears to prolong the activity of serotonin (a neurotransmitter) in the brain. St. John's Wort may also lengthen the performance of dopamine and norepinephrine—two brain chemicals that are linked to depression. In Europe, many doctors prescribe this herb instead of prescription antidepressant drugs.

Note! You can find further details on Stress and Depression by reading my book *"An Easy Way to Understand Stress and Depression"*, which is available from the Kindle Store, or there is a download printable version available at www.wisdomforlifemedia.com.

Thyme

Thyme is often thought of as an herb that is used in the kitchen along with sage, parsley and rosemary. However, it has important medicinal uses, and is often included in over-the-counter mouthwashes and decongestants.

Thyme contains aromatic oil which is an antispasmodic, and is used for digestive problems—by relaxing the smooth muscle tissue of the gastrointestinal tract, as well as being useful for treating bacterial and viral infections. As an expectorant, it is also used for a cough—to loosen and expel phlegm, as well as for laryngitis, sore throat, whooping cough and nervous system disorders.

Additionally, it is used externally as an antiseptic for treating wounds which aids healing.

Una de Gato (Cats Claw)

The bark of a vine from South America. una de gato provides beneficial alkaloids to stimulate the immune system. It is also used for the following:

- In cancer therapy to reduce the side effects of chemotherapy.
- As an anti-inflammatory for all types of arthritis.
- As a bowel and stomach protector and cleanser, and to treat ulcerative colitis as well as stomach ulcers.

- To treat a variety of bowel problems including, but not limited to: Crohn's disease, diverticulitis and irritable bowel syndrome (IBS).

- An excellent general body tonic to tone and protect all body systems.

It is usually taken in capsule form.

Uva Ursi

Uva Ursi is used to treat cystitis—inflammation of the urinary tract. The main component of Uva Ursi is arbutin. Arbutin is absorbed in the stomach where it is converted into a substance with antimicrobial and astringent properties.

Arbutin's main purpose is to soothe irritation and reduce inflammation during urination, as well as to fight infections in the urinary tract.

It is important for the urine to be alkaline for uva ursi to work properly. The acid / alkaline balance (pH) can be determined by using a litmus paper test strip. If the urine is too acidic then it can be brought to an alkaline state by the use of alkalizing agents such as calcium / magnesium supplements, chlorophyll in liquid form (chlorophyll is derived from alfalfa), and by eating alkalizing foods such as tomatoes, and the majority of fruits and vegetables. This is by no means a complete list. Note. While most citrus fruits are acidic, when they have been digested they are alkaline forming.

Acidic foods to avoid would be mainly beef, pork, lamb, butter, peanut butter, and many more. There are some excellent acid / alkaline food lists available on the Internet. Just type "acid alkaline food lists" into your search engine.

Valerian

Valerian Root—a natural plant calcium—is often used as a pain killer. It has been used for centuries to treat anxiety and insomnia, and is best taken before bedtime.

Violet Leaf

Is a good source of vitamin C and beta carotene (which the

body converts to vitamin A as needed). Violet Leaf has antifungal properties in addition to being a diuretic and laxative.

White Willow Bark

The use of White Willow Bark goes back to the time of Hippocrates. This Greek physician wrote about the medicinal benefits of white willow bark in the 5th century B.C.

However, it was in 1829 that scientists in Europe identified salicin as being the active ingredient, which is converted in the body to salicylic acid.

It was used as a popular remedy for the relief of pain in such conditions as inflammation, fever, joint pain and osteoarthritis.

Extracting salicin from herbs was a time consuming process, so in 1852, German scientists developed a synthetic form of salicylic acid. Unfortunately this had a tendency to cause stomach ulcers and bleeding.

Eventually the German company Bayer developed a synthetic version being less harsh which they called acetylsalicylic acid (ASA). This was then manufactured under the trade name aspirin. Today, low dose soluble aspirin is recommended by doctors to reduce a person's risk of a heart attack or stroke by 50 percent. However, aspirin still has the stigma of being associated with causing stomach bleeding and irritating the stomach lining.

Many people prefer White Willow Bark to aspirin because it does not irritate the stomach lining. Researchers have identified a possible reason for this in that salicin found naturally in white willow bark is only converted to the acid form after it is absorbed by the stomach.

Additionally, there are other active compounds in natural White Willow Bark which are not in the synthetic salicin. And these additional compounds make the natural salicin more effective than the synthetic form.

Wild Cherry

Wild Cherry contains a volatile oil which makes it a useful expectorant in cases of excess catarrh, phlegm and bronchitis, colds, cough and asthma. It also has a mild sedative action.

Wild Cherry Supports the digestive system, and is often used as a tonic after an illness to benefit all the body systems.

Wild Yam

Wild Yam supports the glandular system, and is used by pregnant women as a treatment for nausea, to help reduce cramps in later stages of pregnancy, and to help prevent a miscarriage.

It helps support the nervous system and helps reduce the pain associated with gallstones.

Witch Hazel

Witch Hazel has excellent anti-inflammatory and antiseptic properties. It has a high flavonoid content which helps to heal damaged blood vessels.

Yarrow

Yarrow has many uses in herbal medicine. It is often used for wound healing due to the various chemicals contained within the plant. It is used as an antiseptic to kill bacteria, for blood clotting, and as an anti-inflammatory and pain reliever.

Yarrow also supports the digestive system as it contains a chemical similar to chamomile which helps relax the smooth muscle tissue of the digestive tract.

It helps support the glandular system, and has a useful role to play as a sedative.

Yellow Dock

Assists with elimination and is one of the best blood builders in the herbal arsenal.

Yerba Mate

A herb from South America which is used to boost energy and stamina, but unlike caffeine containing plants, Yerba Mate does not cause the jitters or shakes. Historically it has also been used to treat asthma and various allergies.

It is usually made into a tea by pouring hot water on to the leaves, and then it is left for 10 minutes before straining.

Yerba Santa

Yerba Santa is best known as a treatment for bronchial congestion in the chest area, due to its decongestant action. It also supports the digestive system by promoting digestive secretions.

Yohimbe

A native to the Congo, Cameroon, Nigeria, and Gabon, Yohimbe is used to prevent depression as it inhibits monoamine oxidase (MAO) which is a chemical formed in the brain. Additionally it is used to treat erectile dysfunction either as a single herb, or in combination with other herbs.

Yucca Root

Yucca Root is high in fiber content and as such, is an excellent herb for digestive and intestinal problems. It can rid the body of undigested waste toxins which reside in the colon and cause foul smelling gasses.

Historically, Yucca Root has been used as an anti-inflammatory and laxative agent that purges toxins from joints which if left untreated, can cause inflammation that then leads to joint problems such as arthritis. Yucca is also effective at eliminating toxins from the blood, kidneys, liver and lymph.

Consult Your Doctor or a Naturopathic Doctor

In the A-Z of Herbs section I have given a short description of various herbal products that have been used historically by herbalists and naturopaths for many years, but no suggested dosage requirements, or contra-indications.

The reason for this is that everyone is different. One person may need more of a particular product than the next person. Also, a particular product may suit one person, but not another.

Therefore I feel it is extremely important that you consult your doctor or a naturopathic doctor before commencing any supplement or herbal program, or changing your diet.

Additionally, you may be taking prescription medications for various health conditions which will, or could, have a negative impact on your health if you introduce vitamin or mineral supplements or a herbal program. Never take chances with your health.

I know that many doctors are not supportive of using a natural traditional route for health care. If your doctor feels this way and you would like to consider a more natural approach, then change your doctor and find one who is more supportive to your requirements.

About The Author

Brian B Jacques started in business when he was 11 years old, and over the ensuing years, he has developed several very successful businesses. But his main interest for the past 35 years has been in natural health research and book publishing.

He is a founding partner in Nature's Direct LLC a Florida, USA based supplier of nutritional supplements and herbal products, and Wisdom For Life Media, an online publisher of books which focus on the Health, Motivation and Personal Development fields. This company is also based in Florida, USA.

Brian has presented seminars worldwide on such diverse subjects as Health Related issues, Motivation and Personal Development. In addition he has written numerous books, newsletters and articles on these subjects.

His very popular series of Mini Health Books has circulated widely around the world, and many more titles are in preparation.

Brian is a highly motivated individual, so much so that in 1985 he received a UK Industrial Society award for his work in the Motivation and Personal Development fields.

Brian has the following mottos:

- If something does not work out for you, then don't give up, but keep trying, trying, trying until finally you succeed.
- Success or failure in any endeavor is in your own hands.

Brian was born in the UK and lives with his wife in Florida, USA, and East Yorkshire, UK.

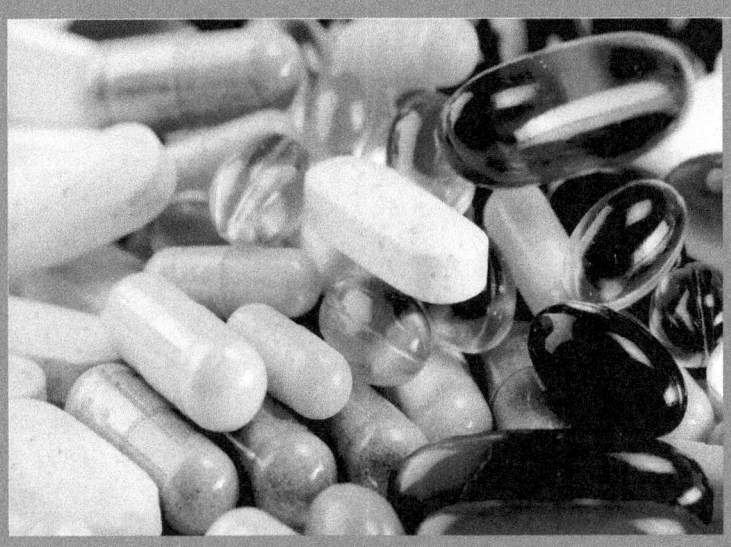

Index

www.ingramcontent.com/pod-product-compliance
Lightning Source LLC
Chambersburg PA
CBHW070459290526
45790CB00003B/1017